SUPER FIT COOKBOOK

PERFECTS FOR BODY-BUILDING

Tyler E. Stoneburner

Contents

Chapter One

INTRODUCTION

Consider whether or not eating like a caveman will help you identify with the Paleo culture. Alternatively, you may blame your weight loss problems on carbs and put yourself through a rigorous ketogenic diet experiment. In other words, you could get lost in the bogs of pure pseudoscience like "cleanses," "unclogging hormones," and other such nonsense.

It's possible to waste months of your life like this, hopping from one diet to the next, with little to show for it at the gym or on the mirror. Then you'll just keep going on your search to find the diet that would finally give you the body you've always wanted, like many others.

Unfortunately, there isn't a single diet that works for everyone. "Shredding" is not a "shortcut." No "weight loss foods" or "muscle-building tips" are available.

"The truth about dieting" is actually quite boring. Millions of books and millions of supplements won't be sold because of it. What it does have is functionality. Efficiently. Unquestionably. Invariably.

What is the reality of this statement?

It can be visualised as a declining importance pyramid with numerous stages, like follows:

BALANCE YOUR ENERGY

Because energy balance is the underlying principle of dieting, it's at the bottom. This is the most important factor affecting your weight increase and loss.

But what exactly is an energy balance?

The link between the amount of energy you use and the amount of energy you produce is known as energy balance. As you may have guessed, kilocalories are used to measure this.

When it comes to weight loss and weight growth (fat and muscle), the basic line is that you must expend more energy than you consume in order to lose weight, and you must consume more energy than you spend in order to gain weight.

To those shaking their heads and thinking I'm drinking decades-old Kool-Aid, here's a question:

Countless meta-analyses and systematic reviews from the previous century all come to the same conclusion: significant weight loss requires energy expenditure to surpass energy intake.

Since the time of Sandow to Reeves and beyond, bodybuilders have used this knowledge to lower and increase their body fat levels on a regular basis.

And why are there always new “calorie-denying” products that fail to acquire traction in the weight reduction community?

Bottom line: a century of metabolic research has conclusively demonstrated the fundamental role that energy balance plays in regulating fat storage and decrease through thermodynamics.

Balance of macronutrients in the body

Macronutrient balance is the next step in the nutrition pyramid.

The dictionary defines macronutrient as “any of the nutritional components of the diet that are required in relatively significant amounts: protein, carbohydrate, fat, and minerals like calcium, zinc, iron, magnesium, and phosphorous.”

In terms of energy balance and weight loss and gain, it’s true that “a calorie is a calorie,” but when it comes to body composition it’s not so simple.

What if I’m wrong?

There is no denying that Professor Mark Haub, who lost 27 pounds on a diet of Twinkies and Doritos along with a few other junk food items like Oreos and Little Debbie snacks, could accomplish the same if he wanted to.

But gaining and losing weight isn't all we're after.

We have a more specific objective in mind: we want to increase our muscle mass while decreasing our fat mass. In order to achieve these objectives, we must keep track of more than simply calories. Additionally, we need to keep an eye on our macro-nutrient consumption.

You need to monitor protein closely if you want to go beyond "weight reduction" and learn how to improve your body composition.

WHICH AMOUNT OF PROTEIN SHOULD YOU BE Eating?

Primary building blocks for the body are proteins. Muscle, tendons, organs, and skin, as well as numerous other molecules essential to life, such as hormones, enzymes and various brain chemicals are all made from them.

Amino acids, the smaller molecules that make up proteins, are connected in a long chain and can take on various shapes.

The human body can manufacture twelve of the amino acids needed to make protein molecules, but we must obtain the other nine from the protein in the food we consume. They're both referred to as “non-essential amino acids,” but only the second group is.

As a general rule, the amount of protein you consume is the most important element in determining whether or not your body is getting enough necessary amino acids.

Although plant-based protein sources like rice and peas have a higher concentration of necessary amino acids than animal-based protein sources like meat and fish, they are not as popular with athletes.

Vegans and vegetarians can acquire enough amino acid-rich protein to build muscle and strength if they organise their meals creatively enough.

It’s fine to vary your carbohydrate and fat consumption as long as you’re not depriving yourself of the essential macronutrient protein.

You’ll lose a lot of muscle if you eat too little protein while lowering your calorie intake for fat loss.

It is also possible to overeat calories in order to gain weight, but not enough protein will result in a decrease in the amount of muscle growth.

This is why “bulking” gets a negative reputation. When done incorrectly, it leads to fat gain rather than muscle gain, which is ultimately detrimental.

What's the problem with too little protein?

For those who routinely exercise, here's what it boils down to for those who are concerned about their health:

If you're not trying to lose weight, aim for 0.8 to 1 gramme of protein per pound of body weight per day if you're lean.

If you're in good shape and trying to lose weight, you should aim for 1 to 1.2 grammes of protein per pound of body weight every day. For fat loss, you'll need more protein if you're slimmer than you are now, according to research. 5

Your protein intake should be set at 1 to 1.2 grammes per pound of lean mass per day if you are obese (25 percent body fat and above in men and 35 percent and more in women).

Why isn't a high-protein diet harmful, you ask? "But wait," you say.

High-protein diets are frequently accused of causing kidney damage and increasing cancer and osteoporosis risk, although these claims are unsubstantiated by scientific evidence.

However, a high-protein diet has never been linked to kidney impairment in healthy persons, only in those who already have renal injury or malfunction.

Even while a high-protein diet is associated with higher blood pressure, it has also been linked to better glucose control in diabetics (particularly when the protein is derived from plants).

This would reduce rather than raise their risk of renal disease.

As a matter of fact, research show that a high-protein diet can really help prevent osteoporosis.

What about the alarming statements that a high-protein diet raises cancer risk and that regular consumption of meat and cheese is as bad for you as tobacco use?

However, despite the fact that this type of sensationalism generates a lot of traffic, it is misleading and scientifically flawed.

The idea that eating protein is comparable to smoking is just sensationalism," he said.

It would have been better if the study's title read, "Excessive protein intake may increase the risk of cancer in persons aged 50 to 65 who had poor diet and lifestyle habits."

We'll discuss meat consumption and health in greater detail later in the book, but here's the bottom line:

A high-protein diet will unquestionably benefit your health, body composition, and performance if you are physically active.

In addition, research reveals that the current RDI (Recommended Daily Intake) of 0.8 grammes per kg of body weight simply isn't enough to maintain lean mass and bone health, therefore avoiding muscle loss and osteoporosis, as they become older.

It's important to know how much carbs you should consume each day.

The low-carbohydrate diet is currently all the rage when it comes to losing weight, but like most diet fads, it falls short of expectations.

Low-carb advocates use roughly 20 research to support their claim that low-carb diets are superior for weight loss.

Low-carb dieting appears to be more effective based on the abstracts of these studies, and this superficial "science" is what most low-carbers rely on to support their ideas.

The difficulty, however, is that many of these studies have a serious flaw in the way they measure protein intake.

There is an issue with these research since the low-carb diets typically had more protein than the low-fat diets.

Yes, one for one... without exception.

What we're truly looking at in these trials is a high-protein, low-carbohydrate diet vs. low-protein, high-fat diet, and the former wins every time.

But we can't overlook the high-protein aspect of the diet and then declare it's more successful because of its low-carb feature.

In fact, better-designed and conducted trials show that low-carb dieting has no specific weight-loss benefits when protein intake is substantial.

What makes protein consumption so crit cal?

Because, as you may be aware, if you don't consume enough protein when dieting to lose weight, you can lose a significant amount of muscle.

11

This obstructs your weight loss in a number of ways:

1. It causes your metabolism to slow down.

12

2. It lowers the number of calories you burn during workouts.

13

3. It interferes with glucose and fat metabolism.14

This is why keeping lean mass should be your top priority when losing weight.

Returning to the "lowcarb diets is better for weight loss" studies stated before, let's look at them again.

In many of these studies, the low-fat groups had less protein than the recommended daily intake, which any nutritionist or personal trainer will tell you is grossly inadequate for weight loss.

In fact, studies show that even doubling or tripling those protein intake amounts isn't enough to totally avoid muscle loss while calorie limiting.

15

So, what happens when you keep protein high and compare high and low carbohydrate levels in terms of weight loss? Is there any research that we can look at?

Yup.

There are four studies that match these requirements that I am aware of, and have a look at them: There is no substantial difference in weight reduction when protein intake is high but carb intake fluctuates. 16

The simple line is that if you consume less calories than you expend while maintaining a high protein intake, you will maximise fat loss while minimising (if not fully avoiding) muscle loss.

Going low-carb won't help you shed any more weight.

HOW MUCH FAT SHOULD YOU EAT ON A DAILY BASIS?

Dietary fats are essential for a range of physiological functions in the body, including cell maintenance, hormone generation, insulin sensitivity, and more.

These processes can be affected if dietary fat intake is too low, which is why the Institute of Medicine recommends that individuals consume 20 to 35 percent of their daily calories from fat.

17

Those percentages, however, were estimated for the average sedentary person, who often eats less than someone who exercises often, especially if that person has a lot of muscle.

A sedentary 190-pound male with a normal amount of lean mass, for example, would burn roughly 2,000 calories per day. According to the Institute of Medicine's studies, he would require 45 to 80 grammes of fat per day. That's logical.

I'm 6′2″ and 191 pounds, and I work out for 4 to 6 hours a week. I'm around 40 pounds stronger than the normal guy my size and weight. As a result, my body burns a lot more calories than my "regular," sedentary counterpart–roughly 1,000 extra calories every day.

My suggested fat intake would climb to 65 to 115 grammes per day if I followed the IoM's advice blindly. But, just because I'm muscular and burn more energy through frequent activity, does my body truly require that much more dietary fat?

It doesn't work that way.

A dietary fat intake of roughly 0.3 grammes per pound of fat-free mass (everything in your body that isn't fat) is all your body requires for its fundamental health needs, according to the nutritional research I've examined.

This equates to around 25% to 35% of your basal metabolic rate (which we'll discuss further later), which is more in line with the IoM's findings.

That's all there is to macronutrient balance. Let's go to the next level of the pyramid.

FOOD OPTIONS

These days, the "clean eating" craze is more prevalent than ever.

While I believe in eating healthy ("clean") foods to provide our bodies with important vitamins and minerals, I also believe that eating only these foods will not result in muscle gain or fat loss.

You can be the world's healthiest eater and still be frail and "skinny-fat."

The reason for this is that when it comes to body composition, how much you eat is more significant than what you eat.

Claiming that one cuisine is “better” than another for weight loss or gain is deceptive since it fails to see the forest for the trees.

Foods have no particular qualities that make them better or worse for losing or gaining weight.

They do, however, have different levels of potential energy (measured in calories) and different macronutrient compositions.

Certain foods are more ideal for losing or gaining weight than others due to these two factors: the calories in foods and how those calories break down into protein, carbohydrate, and fat.

You can lose weight eating whatever you like as long as you limit your calorie intake and maintain a state of negative energy balance, as Professor Haub demonstrated before and as the “If It Fits Your Macros” folks will not stop up about.

However, due to their volume, calorie density, and macronutrient breakdown, certain foods make it easier or harder to lose or gain weight.

In general, foods that are “excellent” for weight loss are those that have a low calorie count but a large volume (and thus satiating).

Lean meats, whole grains, a variety of fruits and vegetables, and low-fat dairy are examples of such foods. These meals are also high in micronutrients, which is very important when your calorie intake is limited.

You can acquire vitamin and mineral deficiencies if you eat too much junk on a calorie-restricted diet.

Foods that promote weight gain are high in calories but low in volume and satiation.

High-calorie beverages (soda, alcohol, fruit juice), candy, and other sugar-laden treats are among these foods. However, many “healthy” foods, such as oils, bacon, butter, low-fiber fruits, and whole-fat dairy products, fall into this group as well. The more calorie-dense, low-satisfaction meals we include in our meal plans, the more likely we are to become hungry and overeat.

Consider it this way: whether you’re trying to lose weight or grow muscle, you can only “afford” so many calories per day, and you have to be careful how you “spend” them.

You want to spend the bulk of your calories on meals that allow you to meet your daily macro- and micronutrient needs without “overdrawing” your energy balance “account” when dieting for fat loss. (I know, this financial metaphor is getting out of hand, but bear with me.)

When you're dieting for muscle gain, you have a lot more calories to burn each day. This makes it easy to meet your macronutrient and micronutrient goals while still having calories left over to spend on, well, whatever you want.

Don't get the wrong idea: I'm not advocating for eating healthy foods in this area. People who try to prove that you can "eat garbage and become shredded" don't have my support. More important than getting incredibly thin while eating boxes of Pop Tarts every week is long-term health.

Instead, here's my rule of thumb: split the money 80-20.

If you consume the majority of your calories (80%) from relatively unprocessed, nutrient-dense foods, you can indulge in your favourite dietary sins while remaining healthy, muscular, and lean.

TIME TO EAT NUTRIENTS

Nutrient timing is at the bottom of the pyramid and is of the least importance.

The short version is that it doesn't really matter when or how often you eat.

Increasing the number of meals you eat does not speed up your metabolism.

19 Carbohydrates eaten late at night do not make you fat. 20 The "anabolic window" after an exercise is more fantasy than actuality. 21

One of our bodies' many virtues is their incredible ability to adapt to the demands we impose on them. You have a lot of leeway here at the top if you get the other sections of the pyramid right—proper energy balance, adequate macronutrient breakdown, and wise meal selections.

You have the option of eating three or thirteen meals per day. Breakfast, dinner, or after your workout are all good times to eat 80 percent of your carbohydrates. After a workout, you're not on the clock and gradually lose the fruits of your labour until you drink a shake.

AT THE END OF THE DAY

If you've been looking for a diet that genuinely works, doesn't make you a slave to arbitrary rules and limits, and is pleasurable enough to be a lifestyle rather than a chore, you've found it.

You'll never go back if you learn how to manipulate energy balance, keep protein consumption high while adjusting carbohydrate and fat intake to match your needs and preferences, consume a wide variety of nutritious foods "supplemented" with certain indulgences, and eat on a schedule that works for you.

SYNOPSIS OF THE CHAPTER

A century of metabolic research has established beyond a doubt that the underlying process that regulates fat store and reduction is energy balance, acting in accordance with the first law of thermodynamics.

You'll lose a lot of muscle if you eat too little protein while lowering your calorie intake for fat loss.

You'll build less muscle if you eat too little protein and a lot of calories to optimum muscle growth.

If you're not trying to lose weight, aim for 0.8 to 1 gramme of protein per pound of body weight per day if you're lean.

If you're in good shape and trying to lose weight, you should aim for 1 to 1.2 grammes of protein per pound of body weight every day.

Prioritize fat loss and protein consumption of 1 to 1.2 grammes of lean mass per pound of lean mass per day for those who are overweight or obese.

Maintaining a calorie deficit and eating plenty of protein will help you shed fat while still keeping musc.e mass. To add to that, going low-carb is not going to help you lose any more weight.

There isn't anything about foods that makes them better or worse for losing or gaining weight.

When it comes to weight loss, foods with low calorie counts but large volume tend to be considered "excellent" (and thus satiating).

In contrast, foods that promote weight gain are low in calories and high in volume and satiety. Many "healthy" foods, such as oils, bacon, butter, low-fiber fruits, and whole-fat dairy products, fit into this category, as do caloric beverages, candy, and other sugar-laden treats.

You can eat as many as thirteen meals a day if you choose. Breakfast, dinner, or after a workout are all acceptable times to consume 80 percent of your daily carbohydrate requirements. After a workout, you don't have to worry about losing your gains until you drink a shake.

Eating protein after an exercise has been shown to be beneficial for muscle building in the long run.

Chapter Two

WHY FLEXIBLE DIETING IS THE BEST PATH TO A PERFECT BODY

There are "pennies of self-esteem" in small victories. King, Florence

I get it if you're dreading the prospect of going on a diet. Most diets feel more like a kind of punishment than a way to enhance one's health.

Most diet "gurus" resort to scare tactics and food restriction instead of teaching you how your metabolism works and providing you with the skills you need to effectively regulate it.

They believe that if you want to lose weight or gain "lean muscle," you should give up almost everything you enjoy eating.

Processed food and refined carbohydrates (like those found in granola) as well as high-glycemic foods (such those in red meat and processed meals) must all be eliminated from the diet.

Everything you own. Put them all in the blazing furnace.

When you eat the same meals every day, seven days a week, it's possible to drastically change your physique without having to give up your favourite foods.

What if, instead of depriving yourself and starving yourself to gain muscle and reduce fat, you simply followed a few flexible dietary guidelines?

How would you like it if I told you that you could ditch dieting's negative connotations and learn to appreciate it instead?

You think it's a scam? Downrightheresy?

That's correct, by the way. When I was a kid, I had the same thoughts. The truth has finally come out, and in this chapter, I'll explain it all to you.

Why Flexible Dieting Is Not a "DIET"

What's the point of a "diet" if you're allowed to eat everything you want? How can you expect to lose weight if you eat a diet high in carbohydrates? Which "dieter" worth his or her salt would dare to indulge in sweets without feeling guilty?

Some of the common complaints of flexible diets include the following. That it is commonly referred to as the "anti-diet" is also demonstrated.

The fact that flexible dieting has different connotations for different people is a major source of contention. It can be utilised for good or evil, much like a superpower.

So, in order to avoid leaving anything out, let's start with a basic blueprint for dieting with flexibility. It everything works out like this:

What you eat is secondary to how much you eat.

If you have certain goals, tastes, and lifestyle, you should customise your daily food intake to those needs.

Give yourself a break. Remain calm and go on.

The key to long-term progress is a culture of long-term compliance.

It is possible to adapt your body's basic energy and nutrient requirements into a diet that you truly enjoy, according to the concept of flexible dieting.

Foods that you enjoy should not be restricted.

Eat when and how you want to, as long as it works for you.

Dieting should be viewed as a way of life, not a short remedy.

Accept your mistakes and get back on the horse with a cool demeanour.

In flexible dieting, these are the tenets of conduct. Because they work, they're becoming increasingly popular.

Theoretically, that's all fine, but you're probably wondering how it'll actually work out. Let's find out what's going on.

WHAT RESULTS FROM A FLEXIBLE DIET

With these considerations in mind, let's look at each of the specifics of how flexible dieting works.

More important than what you eat is how much you eat.

In fact, "clean eaters" have the correct intentions, but their diet philosophy isn't focused on fat loss or muscle growth.

Eating a balanced diet rich in vitamins, minerals, and other nutrients is critical for good health and long life, however as you may be aware, no meal has the ability to produce weight increase or reduction in a person.

1

"Healthy fats" aren't going to save you, and sugar isn't going to kill you.

The notion of "energy balance," which you learnt about in the last chapter, is critical to understanding these "startling" assertions.

There are two types of weight increase and two types of weight loss: a "negative energy balance," or calorie deficit, and a "positive energy balance."

As a result, in this context, a calorie is only an arbitrary unit of measurement.

You can gain weight even if you eat a lot of “clean” foods, like avocado toast.

You can lose weight by adopting a “gas station diet” that consists of the most nutritionally devoid junk you can locate while maintaining a calorie deficit.

BUILD A DIET AND A LIFE STYLE BASED ON THE FOODS YOU ENJOY.

It’s important to eat meals you enjoy. I eat breakfast, lunch, and dinner. 365 days a year. As long as you’re alive.

That is, in fact, correct.

In other words, you won’t be limited to “healthy” options like fruits, vegetables, nuts, and seeds.

It’s best to receive most of your calories from these types of meals in order to maximise health, lifespan, and overall well-being.” That’s correct.

It’s only once you’ve done that, though, that you’ve “earned” the right to indulge in foods that have traditionally been considered “unhealthy,” such as pizza, pastas, cereals, bagels, and fries.

My “daily indulgences” include ice cream, chocolate, muffins, pancakes with syrup, and cookies, just to name a few. There is no hard and fast rule on how many calories I can "afford" to consume.

It doesn't matter if you're trying to lose weight or gain muscle.

Flexible diets can help you get the body and health you desire if you follow the guidelines outlined above.

My words are based on personal experience, not speculation. I keep my body in shape by following my own advice:

Exactly as outlined in this chapter, flexible diets.

Weightlifting for four to six hours a week.

High-intensity interval training (HIIT) is done once a week.

Taking vitamins the right way.

It's done.

Every day, I eat a variety of things that are "supposed" to make me fat and unhealthy, such as grains, dairy, and sugar, along with numerous servings of fruits, vegetables, and high-quality proteins.

The most important thing is to strike a balance. As long as you consume more healthy foods and engage in regular resistance training, you're golden.

"KEEP CALM AND CARRY ON" WITH YOUR DIETARY LAPSES,

Cravings are a common side effect of extremely low-calorie diets. As a result of cravings, "cheating" occurs. Binge-eating is a result of cheating. Furthermore, overeating can lead to a desire to stop altogether.

Does this sound familiar to you? It ought to. Millions of people fall victim to conventional dieting's slick slope every year.

This pattern can be broken with the use of flexible dieting.

You can achieve dietary "magic" when you eat meals that you enjoy, balance your macronutrient intake, and somewhat restrict your calories. You no longer have to contend with the stomach demons clamouring for more food, which is a huge psychological relief.

The process of slimming down becomes much simpler. It's even enjoyable.

However, this does not guarantee that you will never make a mistake. Take it in stride if you find yourself more peckish than usual. Having a difficult week at work or attending social gatherings makes it simple to overeat.

Your daily caloric deficit was effectively reduced to half after you had two scoops of ice cream, so you did not overeat. That's all.

In other words, you went a step further and overate for a few days, which resulted in a small increase in body fat.

What have you done to yourself? Is it just a few days or a few weeks? Even for a week?

"Who cares?" Carry on as if nothing had happened.

As you might expect, even a moderate weekend binge does not necessarily result in a significant increase in body fat. The "damage" will only take a few days or a week to repair.

That's fine, too. Nothing justifies bingeing on self-loathing or shame.

It's better, in my opinion, to merely prepare for tiny setbacks instead. There are times when you'll consume more than you planned. It's not something to be afraid of.

IS THE KEY TO LONG-TERM SUSTAINABLE IMPROVEMENTS.

In other words, "the best diet is the one you can keep to."

As cliché as it may sound, it holds a lot of truth in it. In order to achieve and maintain your desired weight loss, you must adhere to your diet plan for an extended period of time.

Keep in mind that I'm emphasising long-term effects you can rely on.

That's the ultimate goal. It's not about losing weight quickly on a crash diet and then ballooning back to your old weight... or something even more dreadful.

Flexible diets makes it easy to achieve your body composition goals. It's also a long-term habit, not a "quick cure," because it's so adaptable and can fit into any lifestyle.

HOW TO GET STARTED ON A FLEXIBLE DIET

Now that I've convinced you to give flexible dieting a try, let's get down to business.

To begin, here are a few ground rules:

Get the majority of your daily calories (80% or more) from foods that are relatively unprocessed and nutrient-dense.

Because I'm repeating myself, I'm doing it for your benefit.

Even if you can "meet your macros" by eating junk food, that doesn't mean you should. It is important to remember that your body need a wide range of vitamins and minerals in order to function properly. Let me tell you something: Fruity Pebbles and brownies won't bring you to your goal.

Here's a quick guide to some of my favourite, most nutrient-dense foods:

Kale and spinach are the primary dark-leafy greens, but other options include bell peppers and Brussels sprouts as well as mushrooms and onions. Other options include white and sweet potatoes as well as berries, whole wheat, cheese, and yoghurt.

The possibilities are endless if I so desired. And your list may look completely different as a result.. But you get the gist of it...

Get in the habit of eating according to your personal preferences and lifestyle.

It is important to remember that the time of day you take your food is irrelevant.

Meal timing and frequency aren't going to help or hurt your outcomes if you're managing your energy and macronutrient balances correctly.

But if you are serious about weightlifting and gaining muscle mass, you should know that consuming protein and carbs immediately following resistance training will speed up the process of muscle building.

2

It's important to ingest 30 to 40 grammes of protein before and after your exercises, if you routinely lift weights.

When it comes to carbohydrate intake, 30 to 50 grammes before an exercise is ideal, and 1 gramme of carbs for every kilo of body weight is adequate after a workout.

INSTRUCTIONS FOR CREATING A FLEXIBLE DIET PLAN

Surely you've figured out that flexible dieting has a lot to offer. Dieting has never been so simple as it is with this strategy.

Fat loss and muscle gain are the primary objectives here.

FAST AND EASY WAYS TO LOSE WEIGHT

Maintaining a long-term calorie deficit is the key to fat loss, as you know. So, the first step is to determine how many calories you should be consuming each day to achieve your weight loss goals.

Your body needs a specific quantity of energy in order to maintain its own functions. You require a constant supply of fuel for your body's cells, and this fuel comes from the food you eat.

For a 24-hour period, your basal metabolic rate, or BMR, measures how much energy your body consumes to accomplish the essential tasks linked to your survival (excluding any and all physical activity).

This is what we mean when we use the word "basal." "The physical and chemical processes in an organism by which it produces, maintains and destroys material substances and by which it makes energy accessible" is the definition of metabolism, which is metabolic.

Long-term food and activity patterns can influence basal metabolic rate (a process known as "metabolic adaptation" and an interesting one in and of itself), but a formula like the Katch McArdle can accurately predict BMR for the majority of people with high precision.

As you can see, here's the process:

In other words, the BMR is 370 plus (21.6 * LBM).

In this calculation, the term “lean body mass” (LBM) is used to refer to the nonfat components of the human body.

LBM is calculated by subtracting your body fat weight from your total body weight, resulting in the weight of everything save your body fat.

Here’s a peek at it:

LBM is equal to the sum of one’s lean body mass and one’s body fat percentage (represented as a decimal number).

For example, if I weigh 191 pounds and have an 8 percent body fat percentage, my LBM would be as follows:

If 1 is subtracted from 0, the result is 176 lb (LBM)

Since one kilogramme weighs 2.2 pounds, the following calculation can be used to get my basal metabolic rate:

There are approximately 2,098 calories in a pound of beef.

There is no clear answer to how much energy your body burns when you are at rest, however this BMR calculation is fairly correct for the vast majority of individuals

TDEE, or “total daily energy expenditure,” is the metric you use to estimate how much additional energy you burn through physical exercise.

In a 24-hour period, this is the entire amount of energy that your body expends, and it changes daily (some days you move more and some days less).

To find your TDEE, multiply your BMR using the following formula:

As long as you work out for one to three hours every week.

You'll get to 1.35 if you work out 4 to 6 hours a week.

For those who work out intensely for six or more hours a week, this increases by 1.5.

The entire amount of energy your body expends on a daily basis can be calculated using this number.

Your weight would stay about the same if you consumed that many calories every day. In order to lose weight, you must cut back on your caloric intake... the answer to this question depends on how much less.

Calculate the calorie deficit you'll need to meet.

A calorie deficit of 20 to 25 percent is a good starting point for fat loss. Anything larger can create unpleasant side effects associated with "starvation dieting."

As a result, your daily caloric intake should be set at 75% to 80% of your calculated total daily energy expenditures (TDEE).

For example, my usual daily TDEE is roughly 3,000 calories, therefore when I want to lose weight, I put my intake at about 2,300 calories.

Set macronutrient goals for yourself

It is now time to convert your calorie aim into a protein, carbohydrate, and fat target.

What you need to know:

To maintain a healthy weight, eat 1.2 grammes of protein per pound of body weight for men and women.

If you're overweight, consume 1 gramme of protein for every pound of lean body mass you have.

Consume 0.2 grammes of fat per pound of body weight. "

Carbohydrates provide the remainder of your caloric intake.

For me, the following is how it unfolds:

A person's weight is 191.

Consumption of 2,300 calories per day

920 calories Equals 230 grammes of protein (1 gramme of protein is approximately 4 calories)

360 calories come from 40 grammes of fat (1 gramme of carbohydrate is also approximately 4 calories)

1020 calories = 255 grammes of carbs (1 gramme of fat is approximately 9 calories)

It's now time to transform your figures into a meal plan that you'll look forward to eating.

To begin, prepare a list of things you'd like to eat on a daily basis and look up the macronutrient profiles of those meals, Excel is a popular tool for this, with columns for protein, carbohydrate, fat, and calorie content for each food listed side-by-side.

Using these foods, begin putting together meals until your total daily calorie consumption falls within 50 calories of your aim.

Once you've made a strategy, you'll stick to it every single day of your life. If you get bored with a particular snack or meal along the road, simply swap it out for something else you prefer and that satisfies your calorie requirements.

It's as easy as that!

Flexibility in Dieting for Muscle Building

Eating less than your TDEE is the key to fat loss. You consume a little more when you want to build muscle.

You should eat roughly 10% more than your usual TDEE if you want to maximise muscle growth. To maximise growth, you need a small amount of extra calories.

For "bulking," the macronutrient breakdown is also different:

A pound of body weight in protein is about one gramme of protein per serving.

Amount of fat you should consume depends on your weight.

Carbohydrates provide the remainder of your caloric intake.

In other words, here's what it means to me (and I've rounded the numbers to make things easier):

760 calories are in 190 grammes of protein.

540 calories come from 60 grammes of fat.

2,000 calories = 500 grammes of carbohydrate

CALORIE COUNTING DOESN'T APPEAR TO WORK FOR EVERYONE, FOR SOME REASON

Counting calories can be difficult for a variety of reasons. Here are the most common ones I've encountered in my work with hundreds of clients who are trying to gain muscle and lose fat.

To many, the idea of having to plan and track what they eat is a huge turn-off.

Others find meal planning and calculating calories with My Fitness Pal to be a mental strain.

Unplanned meals cooked by others, which are difficult to assess in terms of calories, are a common lifestyle for many people.

After seeing how easy it is to lose weight with calorie tracking and a flexible diet, most of these people, in my opinion, will never go back.

No more wishing and hoping that this would be the diet that finally works as a result of having to make the necessary adjustments, but the benefits far outweigh any inconvenience.

They despise the thought of being forced to limit their food intake in any way.

People's relationships with food can be peculiar, to say the least.

Rather than feeling like a "slave" to the calorie count, they want to be able to eat anything they want whenever they want.

Change is more difficult for these people, in my experience. Fad diets, cleanses, and weight loss medicines are just some of the things they attempt before finally surrendering to the master of energy balance and choosing to stay fat rather than count a calorie.

Regularly, they overeat.

Of course, this happens all the time.

A couple more bites during breakfast...

a second helping of salad dressing for lunch...

a little unplanned dessert at dinner.

These "little" portions of extra calories might easily negate the moderate calorie deficit you are seeking to sustain on a regular basis.

The answer is simple: Plan or track everything that goes into your mouth on a daily basis.

They don't weigh and measure their food properly.

This is an unintentional reversal of the original error. Many people overeat without even realising it because they use sloppy methods of meal measurement.

My oatmeal, for example, has 300 calories in a dry cup, according to the nutrition facts panel. I'm tempted, so I pull out my measuring cup, add 300 calories, and record it as a "slightly heaping" cup. But I'm wrong: Oatmeal has a calorie count of slightly over 360.

Human mistake is what got me in a bind here. It's possible to over or undershoot the "one cup" mark.

I should have weighed the oats in grammes instead of measuring it out by the cup. A serving of dry oats that weighs eighty grammes contains around 300 calories.

As a result, I overdo by about 50 calories in that meal, but life continues on. ′

I'm craving peanut butter a few hours later, so I consume two tablespoons, which is 188 calories, according to the package's nutrition information. I take a spoon and fill it to just above the rim with delicious nut butter, which I taste with gusto.

Because 32 grammes of peanut butter has 188 calories in it, my haphazard scooping resulted in 40 grammes, which had an additional 238, making the total calorie count 235.

It doesn't take me long to make the same error several more times with my ketchup at dinner, cream in my latte, and chocolate squares for dessert, and I've successfully erased my calorie deficit for the day.

They are as dishonest as a professional eater.

Having a moderate cheat meal once a week while on a diet is a good idea.

An added benefit is that it may help you maintain your weight loss, depending on your body fat percentage at the time.

It's important to note that I only mentioned one rather indulgent meal. To avoid undoing a week's worth of fat loss, do not have a cheat day or an all-out binge meal. (Alcohol and greasy foods are the worst combination.)

It's fine to have an extra few hundred calories in your daily calorie intake while you're on a cheat day, but don't go overboard.

You can even lower your daily carbohydrate and fat intake if necessary in order to "store up" calories for the larger meal and therefore keep your daily caloric intake within a reasonable range.

TDEE is calculated inaccurately by these individuals.

Because the activity multipliers in scientific formulas often used to compute TDEE are just too high, this is a very simple mistake to make. Most bodybuilders are aware of this, but most “laymen” aren’t.

The activity multipliers I provide in this book are, therefore, smaller than those found in most calorie calculators, for the same reason.

It is necessary to “correct” their metabolisms.

It’s common knowledge that the most effective way to lose weight is to drastically cut caloric intake while simultaneously increasing energy expenditure over the course of a typical week.

For the time being, this strategy will work, but it will eventually fail.

Why?

As a result of your body becoming accustomed to the amount of energy you provide it with. Energy intake and output must be balanced in order for it to be effective (to erase your calorie deficit).

To put it another way, a person's metabolism naturally slows down when they're attempting to lose weight (burning less energy).

3 Down-regulation occurs more quickly and intensely if you decrease your caloric intake. 4

There is a decrease in the amount of impulsive behaviour, such as wandering around while talking on the phone, hopping from one restroom to another, drumming your fingers on the table while reading, or bobbing your knees when you're thinking.

5

Non-exercise activity thermogenesis, or NEAT, is the term for the energy used in these activities, and it accounts for a higher portion of daily energy expenditure than most people think.

NEAT might vary by up to 2,000 calories a day among individuals, according to research.

6 Taking the stairs whenever possible, wa king small distances instead of driving, doing some tasks instead of watching TV, and so on, could help people burn an additional 350 calories each day, according to the same research.

Another consideration is the amount of energy expended during exercise.

To put it another way, it follows that if you lose weight, the amount of energy you use when exercising is also reduced (it costs more energy to move a heavier body). According to studies, this is indeed the case. 7

When reducing calories for weight loss, energy expenditure is lower than normal even if the body weight is artificially boosted by a weight vest, according to studies.

8

To summarise, the body has a variety of mechanisms for reducing energy use and ensuring that dietary intake is in sync with metabolic output. Then, even if you're eating a very low-calorie diet and exercising a lot, you may not see any weight loss.

For many people, the only way to get out of this situation is by reducing their caloric intake or exercising more, which only results in more metabolic slowdown.

This might spiral out of control.

"Reverse dieting" is a term used to describe the process of substantially and continuously reducing one's metabolic rate, which is commonly referred to as metabolic "adaptation" or even "damage."

When someone writes to me and complains that they haven't lost weight, I always want to know what exactly is going on.

If not, why aren't they dropping pounds? What's the latest on how long this has gone on? Do you think they've lost weight? Is their stomach getting flatter (a sure sign of weight loss)?

Most of the time, the responses I get go something like this:

How about 1 pound a week? Isn't that more than enough??" In other words, "I haven't dropped any weight in the last four days," "I can't see my abs yet," and so on.

It's important to note that these folks are frequently making good progress toward their weight loss objectives, but they have unreasonable, unreachable criteria in place.

Big fitness websites and major network reality shows are often fueling standards that are often fueled by ludicrous, false 2- and 3-month transformations portrayed on these websites.

You're doing well if you're shedding one pound every seven to ten days. You can't stop now.

However, if your weight remains stable after seven to ten days, you need to either increase your activity level or decrease your caloric intake.

They put too much emphasis on the weight.

Even though the scale is definitely trending in the right direction, it isn't the final word.

Lifting weights is not recommended for beginners, as this will result in a rise in body weight due to muscle gain (yes, you can gain muscle while losing fat), as well as an increase in glycogen (a carbohydrate your body needs for energy) and water storage in the muscles you are exercising.

They may wonder why their jeans fit looser and they look thinner yet their weight hasn't changed at all if they don't realise this.

Simply put, the weight gained from muscle is "replacing" the fat that was lost.

Make sure you focus on your body composition rather than just your weight when it comes to this situation. We're looking for gains in lean muscle mass and a decrease in body fat percentage, which can be more properly determined by looking in the mirror or measuring your waist circumference.

It's time to make a change if your scale, mirror, and waist measurements have all remained the same for seven to ten days.

Many people fail or feel like they're failing with calorie counting because of these reasons. Follow the advice in this chapter, and you'll have a lot of success and even enjoy the process.

THE FINAL ANALYSIS

You have every right to be dubious about the efficacy of flexible diets. When I originally came upon it, I thought it was a terrible waste of time, but I rapidly realised otherwise.

You don’t have to give up your favourite foods in order to have a healthy body.

Flexible dieting makes this bold claim, and you’ll see for yourself just how true it is.

Good luck with your “diet”!

Chapter Three

THE HUMAN BODY

If you eat 80% of your calories from foods that are generally unprocessed and nutrient-dense, you can eat 20% of your calories from foods that most diet "gurus" discourage.

You'll eat more than you meant at least once in a while. It's not something to be afraid of.

A calorie deficit of 20 to 25 percent is a good starting point for weight loss. "Starvation dieting" might have unpleasant side effects if you eat too much at once.

Muscle growth can be maximised by eating 10% more than your typical daily energy expenditure.

The moderate calorie deficit you're seeking to sustain each day might be quickly negated if you consume many "small" meals of extra calories.

Even if you're "cheating" by consuming a few hundred extra calories, you shouldn't go overboard.

The human body has a variety of techniques to conserve energy and balance intake and output. Then, even if you're eating a very low-calorie diet and exercising a lot, you may not see any weight loss.

You're doing well if you're shedding one pound every seven to ten days. You can't stop now. However, if your weight remains stable after seven to ten days, you need to either increase your activity level or decrease your caloric intake.

We're looking for gains in lean muscle mass and a decrease in body fat percentage, which can be more properly determined by looking in the mirror or measuring your waist circumference.

Scale, mirror, and waist measurements should alter if they haven't changed in 7 to 10 days.

HOW TO EAT HEALTHY WITHOUT CONSCIOUSLY MONITORING YOUR CALORIES

There is nothing magical about spending more time on something than anybody else might reasonably expect. JONES CHRIS

It's easy to lose weight by tracking your caloric intake, but if your goal is to feel and look good rather than lose weight, you don't need to do it every time you eat.

A healthy body composition allows you to take a more relaxed approach to dieting, relying on wise food choices and your natural appetite.

In this chapter, I'm going to share with you some easy dietary rules that will help you build healthy dietary habits conducive to maintaining a lean physique without having to plan or track everything you eat.

Consume A HEALTHY, HIGH-PROTEIN DIET.

Every few months, a new fad diet that promises to satisfy your hunger pangs appears on television shows, in magazines, and on bestseller lists.

You've heard it all before: weight loss is easy, you'll have endless energy, you'll live forever, and so on and so forth. Depending on who you listen to, things can get a little muddled.

Paleo, Mediterranean, and low-carb diets are only some of the many diets that have been around for a long time, while others, like the current low-carb craze, haven't lived up to their hype and are likely to fade away (the HCG diet and other forms of starvation dieting come to mind).

That being said, the most successful diets all have one thing in common: they require a high protein intake.

Let's take a brief look at the most important advantages of a protein-rich diet.

On a high-protein diet, you build more muscle and become stronger.

It should come as no surprise that a high-protein diet can help you gain muscle more quickly. Strength and muscle go hand in hand.

Training your muscles simultaneously damages and breaks down muscle tissue and begins a process known as "protein synthesis" whereby the body generates (synthesises) new muscle proteins in order to replace and add to the damaged tissues.

Increasing your protein intake through exercise and resistance training is a key reason why you'll build greater muscle and strength.

On a high-protein diet, you lose more fat and less muscle.

When you're trying to lose weight, you're really trying to lose fat.

Research has shown that a high-protein diet is superior for both shedding fat more quickly and retaining muscle.

2 To put it simply, a high-protein diet results in more fat and less muscle being lost.

A high-protein diet is easier to keep to when in a calorie deficit since it causes less mood disturbance, tension, fatigue, and diet dissatisfaction than lower-protein diets, and increased dietary compliance means better fat loss results in the long run. ”

A HIGH-PROTEIN DIET MAKES YOU FEEL FULLER QUICKER.

Hunger is a common dietary problem, especially for those trying to lose weight by cutting calories.

Having a grumbling pit in your stomach all day makes it difficult to keep track of your food consumption, but a high-protein diet can help.

There is research to support the idea that consuming more protein reduces hunger through a variety of mechanisms, including the alteration of hormones associated with hunger and fullness.

Researchers have found that high-protein meals are less likely to lead to overeating than high-fat meals, which means you'll feel filled for longer, reducing the risk of overindulging.

On a high-protein diet, you retain more muscle as you become older.

Sarcopenia, the age-related degenerative loss of muscle, is debilitating and, in the end, life-threatening. More muscle loss with age is associated with an increased risk of death from accident and disease, according to studies. 6

Protein is needed more frequently by the elderly since they are unable to utilise it as well as younger people. Even the elderly can grow muscle with resistance training (yes, sarcopenia can be reversed or even prevented by incorporating a high-protein diet). 7

Osteoporosis, another severe health concern connected with ageing, is similarly reduced by a high-protein diet.

WHICH FOODS ARE HIGH IN PROTEIN AND WHICH ARE NOT?

As you may be aware, the issue of how much protein to consume is not an easy one to answer definitively, although a broad consensus does emerge from the wealth of research available:

0.8 to 1 gramme of protein per pound of body weight is enough to get the many benefits of a high-protein diet if you are relatively thin and not in a calorie deficit.

That's what bodybuilders have believed for decades: 1 gramme of protein per pound of body weight, according to the "gym legend."

Protein intake of 1 to 1.2 grammes per pound of body weight is recommended for people who are in a calorie deficit and are moderately thin.

A growing body of evidence demonstrates that resistance-trained athletes' protein requirements rise as their weight diminishes (the leaner you are, the more protein your body will need to preserve muscle while in a calorie deficit).

For obese people (more than 25% body fat in males and more than 35% in women), 1 gramme of protein for every 1 pound of lean mass is sufficient.

Eat A LOT OF LOW-CALORIE, FIBROUS FOODS.

Fermentable carbohydrates including fruits, legumes, and grains are all sources of fibre, which is an indigestible carbohydrate. Soluble and insoluble fibres are available.

Soluble fibre is a type of fibre that may be dissolved in water and has the effect of slowing digestion.

A study has revealed that bacteria in the colon digest soluble fibre, therefore it has no effect on stool weight.

10 The colon's primary source of fuel, however, is faecal matter, which stimulates the growth of good bacteria and fatty acids. 11

Beans, peas, oats, fruits like plums, bananas, and apples, vegetables like broccoli, sweet potatoes, and carrots, and nuts, with almonds being the most fiber-rich.

Stool weight is increased by insoluble fibre, which does not dissolve in water.

12 Despite the fact that it slams into the walls of the digestive system and inflicts harm, research has proven that this procedure is beneficial. 13

Foods rich in insoluble fibre include whole grains such as brown rice and barley; legumes; vegetables like peas, green beans; avocados; the skins of some fruits such as kiwis and tomatoes; and the skins of some berries, such as pomegranates and cherries.

Most vegetables and some fruits, which are high in water content, are excellent for promoting health and reducing weight gain.

Despite their modest caloric content, they pack a nutritional punch and are a great way to keep track of your daily caloric intake.

Apples, bananas, Brussels sprouts, spinach, and oranges are some of my favourite fibre fruits and vegetables. You can keep both your health and your body composition in check by eating at least 2 to 3 cups of both fruits and vegetables each day, according to the USDA.

REDUCE YOUR CONSUME OF BAD FATS.

In addition to aiding the absorption of other nutrients, fats nourish the nervous system, keep cells intact, and regulate hormone levels, among many other functions.

Fats, on the other hand, are not all created equal. Types can either benefit or hinder your health.

Unrefined plant oils such as olive oil, coconut oil, and peanut oil are good sources of healthy fat. So are butters derived from these oils; dairy products; wild-caught fish; and lean meats from pastured animals fed natural diets are also good sources of healthy fat.

These foods' positive effects on health have been well documented in scientific literature.

Olive oil decreases inflammation in the body, omega-3 fatty acid-rich fish protect the brain from age-related decline, and people who consume the most dairy are less likely to acquire heart disease and diabetes than those who eat the least of it.

14

Foods high in unhealthy fats include processed meats such as low-quality sausage or jerky; fried foods such as donuts and fried chicken; packaged foods such as pastries and breakfast cereal; microwave popcorn; frozen pizza and low-quality yoghurt and peanut butter; and low-quality yoghurt and peanut butter.

Once again, the research shows that these foods are harmful to the body as a whole.

Obesity and many chronic diseases, such as hypertension, heart disease, and cancer, are linked to a diet high in fried foods. Many packaged foods include trans fat, a processed form of fat that has been linked to an increased risk of heart disease, diabetes, infertility, and other health issues. 15

Food manufacturers employ trans fat, a synthetic form of saturated fat, to increase the shelf life of their products and enhance their taste. Unlike the trans fats found in TV meals, trans fats found in meat and dairy products are different.

Hydrogenated and partially hydrogenated oils are the most prevalent sources of trans fats in food (oils that have hydrogen atoms added to them). Trans fats can be found in any food containing "hydrogenated oil" or "partially hydrogenated oil."

Trans fats pose a serious health risk because of how little of them it takes to have a harmful effect. In a study involving more than 120,000 female nurses, the risk of heart disease was doubled if trans fats were substituted for 2 percent of daily calories. 16

Since trans fats are linked to heart disease, the American Heart Association and the Institute of Medicine recommend that you limit your intake of trans fat to less than 2 grammes per day. Personally, I do not eat any items that contain trans fats, and I strongly advise you to do so as well. It's fine to have some now and then, but I wouldn't make it a daily habit.

It's not as simple as looking for goods labelled "trans fat free" to stay away from them. A serving of food must include fewer than 0.5 grammes of "zero grammes trans fat per serving" to fulfil the FDA's definition of "zero grammes trans fat per tablespoon," no more than 7 percent trans fat by weight, or less than one gramme per tablespoon. Manufacturers are allowed to advertise that their product is trans fat-free even if it contains 0.49 grammes of trans fat in a serving.

As long as we're trying to limit our daily trans fat intake to no more than 2 grammes, it's important to be aware of these "false zero" items.

The biopsychology of eating foods high in harmful fats should also be considered while making dietary changes. This can lead to overeating because foods high in harmful fats tend to be both delicious and calorie-dense. 17

See if you can cut back on your consumption of harmful fats. I'm not telling them not to do it. That's because if you eat a mostly balanced diet and consistently exercise, you won't be harmed by occasional indulgences in junk food.

A healthy diet and regular exercise can help you avoid long-term repercussions from occasional “lapses” in your diet and exercise regimen.

FISH, NUTS, AND OILS ARE THE BEST WAY TO GET THE MOST OF YOUR DIETARY FAT.

Unsaturated fat, which is liquid at room temperature, is found in these foods.

Heart health is improved, blood pressure is lowered, and the risk of developing heart disease, stroke, and diabetes is reduced by consuming unsaturated fats.

18

The American Heart Association recommends that you acquire the majority of your daily fat calories from unsaturated fats (i.e. more than 50% of your daily fat calories).

This is a simple process. There are around 12 grammes of unsaturated fats in a tablespoon of olive oil, a handful of almonds provides about 9 grammes, and a 4-ounce plate of salmon delivers about 11 grammes.

KEEP YOUR SATURATED FAT INVOLVEMENT LOWER THAN YOU THINK (LESS THAN 10 percent OF YOUR TOTAL DAILY CALORIES)

People who are concerned about their health should steer clear of these foods because they contain a lot of saturated fat. It's a saturated fat if it is solid at room temperature.

Recent study has cast doubt on the long-held belief that saturated fat raises the risk of heart disease.

19

As a result of numerous diet "gurus" promoting high-fat diets, meat and dairy consumption have witnessed a rebirth.

Researchers in nutrition and cardiology have slammed the research that has been used to support this movement for numerous errors and omission, therefore it is difficult to trust it.

20

There is a substantial correlation between a diet high in saturated fat and heart disease, according to these researchers, who recommend that we stick to the recommended dietary guidelines for saturated fat intake (less than 10% of daily calories).

I don't think it's safe to say that we can eat as much saturated fat as we want and not worry about our health. To be on the safe side, I'll wait for more studies before jumping on board.

Saturated fat consumption can be reduced in a number of simple methods, according to the CDC:

Choose thinner pieces of beef that aren't marbled (i.e. where the fat appears embedded in the meat). Round cuts and sirloin cuts are among the leaner cuts available in the market. Meats should be trimmed of all visible fat before to consumption.

Make sure to remove the skin from chickens before cooking.

Before reheating soups or stews, remove the solid fats from the top.

Low-fat (1 percent) or fat-free (skim) milk should be consumed instead of whole or 2 percent milk, which are higher in fat content.

Shop for low-fat or non-fat versions of your favourite dairy items, such as cheeses and milk.

Snack on a low-fat or fat-free frozen dessert when you're in the mood for something sweet. Saturated fat is frequently absent from these formulations.

Saturated fat should be kept to a minimum in baked goods, breads, and sweets. The Nutrition Facts label provides this information.

At mealtime, pay attention. Saturated fat is found in some convenience foods, such as sandwich crackers. Take a fruit and non-fat or low-fat yoghurt instead.

You don't have to do everything on this list. You can pick and choose what works best for your diet and lifestyle.

Personally, I eat roughly 3,000 calories each day, which implies my saturated fat intake should be around 35 grammes per day (which comprises about 315 calories) (which contains about 315 calories). However, I choose butter over low-fat spreads, and 2 percent milk rather than fat-free milk in my diet.

Reduce your intake of foods that have been overly processed.

In the world of health and nutrition, the term "processed foods" is often used as a villain, but the fact is that nearly every meal you can consume has been processed in some form.

For thousands of years, we've been processing our food, and not all modern ways are harmful. For example, blanching and freezing vegetables preserves both their freshness and their nutritional content. To kill specific bacteria, seeds must be squeezed into oil and milk must be pasteurised.

Other tactics for food processing that may be damaging to our health include the use of preservatives, such as trans fats, to extend the shelf life of food; the addition of huge amounts of salt and sugar to enhance the flavour; and the smoking, curing, salting or adding preservatives of meat.

As you've learned, you don't have to fully avoid foods that have been overprocessed. All you have to do is set a cap on how many you have. You'll be alright if you eat most of your calories from unprocessed foods.

This can be done in a number of ways, including:

Store-bought salad dressings should be avoided at all costs. Make your own from the ground up if you want. Their flavour and nutritional value are unmatched.

Refuse to eat the junk food like chips, pretzels and sugary cereal that is excessively processed and salty. There are better options for snacking, such as fruit, almonds, granola and nut butter.

Remove the non-dairy creamers and stick to goods manufactured with real dairy milk or soy- or nut-milks instead.

Remove light butters and vegetable spreads from your diet. Replace it with normal butter if you want.

Don't drink sodas or fruit juices, please. Instead, hydrate yourself with water. Try adding some fruit like strawberry, lemon, lime, or watermelon to your water if you find it bland.

Keep your freezer stocked with a variety of frozen vegetables and fruits. USDA "U.S. Fancy" items are better quality than "U.S. First" or "Use First 2," which are the USDA's top two grades.

Whole grains are better than white ones. A simple approach to enhance your daily intake of fibre and other nutrients is to switch to whole-grain versions of refined white bread, pasta, and rice.

THE FINAL ANALYSIS

Keeping track of your daily caloric intake and macronutrient intake is the best method to ensure that your weight loss efforts are successful, but if the thought of doing this at every meal for the rest of your life makes you uncomfortable, I understand.

Because of this, you don't need to.

Plan and monitor your food consumption if you want to maximise fat reduction or maintain an extremely low body-fat percentage, just like I do (below 10 percent for men and below 20 percent for women). This is the time when you need to be extremely precise with your calorie intake, as I described in the previous chapter.

If you want to avoid weight gain and stay healthy, follow the advice in this chapter.

Chapter Four

TRADITIONAL VS ORGANIC

DO YOU PREFER TRADITIONAL OR ORGANIC FOOD? SCIENCE-BASED COMMENTS

What does it matter if you're rich or poor when your stomach is full? EURIPEDES

Organic food was a niche business a decade ago, catering to a small segment of the population.

This is one of the most popular food fads today, with many large food producers rapidly developing their organic divisions and the majority of Americans at least occasionally buying organic products.

Is this the latest craze? Yes, organic food costs more, but is it worth it? Is there a significant difference between these and the standard fare?

As for the "non-believers," they contend that the health benefits of eating organic are nothing more than a clever marketing ploy to raise profit margins.

Who is correct?

What Is Organic?

The advantages and downsides of organic food should be discussed before we get into the specifics.

There are no synthetic pesticides, genetically modified organisms (GMOs), petroleum- and sewage sludge-based fertilisers, or irradiation in organic crops.

It's important to note that organic cattle must be raised without the use of antibiotics, growth hormone or animal byproducts, and must have access to the outdoors as well as organic feed.

It's easy to see why organic foods are so popular: their very definition implies that they are better for you. It's reasonable to think that the more natural and less processed a product is, the better it is for us. As with the multivitamin, many people buy organic foods based only on this "faith".

According to labelling, it's this way...

PUT A FOCUS ON THE SEAL.

Organic food must fulfil strict USDA requirements for how it's grown, handled, and processed before it can be sold. A dish that meets these requirements will be marked with the following logo:

However, not all organic food is created equal.

Certified Organic 100% of the time

To use this certification, the product must include only organically grown ingredients, with the exception of salt and water.

Organic

If a product has this designation, it signifies that, except from salt and water, 95% of its contents are organic.

Organic Ingredients are Used in This Recipe

This logo indicates that, aside from salt and water, 70% of the ingredients in a product are organic.

Is eating organic food better for your health?

The widely cited Stanford study which stated that "The published literature lacks compelling evidence that organic foods are much more nutritious than conventional foods" could be used to persuade you that organ c foods are a waste of money.

1

It's not uncommon for individuals to address the issue as if it were a straightforward case on Judge Judy.

There's a lot more to be considered in the scientific examination of organic foods, though, anc this is a poor and deceptive approach.

To begin, some scientists have taken issue with the Stanford study's methodology, which has been accused of cherry-picking papers to support its conclusions and ignoring data that doesn't; using ambiguous terminology; and extending their findings to "answer" questions that it can't.

2

Secondly, if you take the time to analyse the many papers mentioned in the analysis, you will discover that eating organic food has numerous advantages.

The nutritional value of organic crops is higher than that of conventional crops.

For instance, an extensive study found that organic farming yields crops that contain 10% to 30% more nutrients than conventionally grown crops, with higher levels of antioxidants (vitamin C, antioxidants, and phenolic acids), as well as higher levels of protein (vitamin A).

3

When researchers from Newcastle University and a big team of specialists reviewed the same literature as the controversial Stanford University study, they used more rigorous criteria to determine how reliable their findings were and how important they were.

As a result, Stanford researchers concluded that a 10% to 30% increase in nutritional density was not "substantially more nutritious."

An over-simplification of the issue is that persons who follow an average Western diet would benefit from slight increases in certain important nutrients.

4

DECREASE YOUR EXPOSURE TO PESTICIDES WITH ORGANIC CROPS

Pesticide residues in organic crops are 10 to 100 times lower than in conventional crops, according to research.

5 Multiple pesticide residues and high-risk pesticides are extremely rare in organic foods.

Conventional meats contain pesticides and other chemicals, which accumulate in fat tissue, making them a double-edged sword.

6

Pesticide exposure poses an overall health risk, not only the number of residues that we are exposed to.

According to a study, switching from conventional to organic foods reduces pesticide exposure by 94 percent and eliminates high-risk compounds in particular, resulting in a significant reduction in pesticide exposure.

7

Organophosphates, which are commonly used in the farming of conventional crops, have been linked to an increased risk of autism, ADHD, and asthma in children who are exposed to them during pregnancy.

8

These compounds have been proven to raise the likelihood of cognitive impairments, such as a lower IQ, in children.

9

Children who eat an organic diet are less likely to be exposed to pesticides and may have a lower chance of developing antibiotic-resistant infections, according to the American Academy of Pediatrics.

10

LESS ANTIBIOTIC-RESISTANT BACTERIA ARE FOUND IN ORGANIC MEATS.

Research reveals that eating antibiotic-treated meat from animals contributes to human antibiotic resistance, which is a severe public health issue.

11

Essentially, animals that have been treated with antibiotics produce antibiotic-resistant germs that can be passed on to other microorganisms and eventually humans.

12

Using antibiotics to treat organic food animals is prohibited, which is one of the reasons why organic meat has a 66% lower prevalence of bacteria resistant to ampicillin.

13

GROWTH HORMONES MAY BE HARMFUL TO YOUR HEALTH IN ORGANIC MEATS.

Cattle-hormone use has long been linked to health issues for consumers, and the scientific community's worry has only intensified since the 1999 study performed by the EU Scientific Committee on Veterinarian Measures related to Public Health (a mouthful) was published.

14

Research reveals that hormone-treated animals may have a wider range of impacts than previously thought, and the discussion over long-term effects on people is shifting to how big of an influence it has rather than if it has any affect at all.

15

What are the drawbacks of eating organic food?

You may be wondering, "So what's the deal with organic foods?" There are, of course, certain drawbacks.

It is expensive to eat organic food.

There is a price to pay for being entirely organic, so make sure you have enough money in your bank account.

If you have the money to spare, you can't go wrong by exchanging your conventional foods for organic ones.

Choosing organic for some goods while using conventional for others is a great way to maximise your organic budget, but if that isn't an option, we'll go into more detail about this in a moment.

The shelf life of organic foods is significantly less than that of conventionally produced ones.

As a minor detail, organic food spoils more quickly, which means more trips to the store and more wasted food.

This, in turn, raises the price of organic food.

Organic foods can be difficult to find.

In the absence of a Whole Foods in your immediate area, it can be difficult to find an organic food retailer with an extensive assortment.

Organic food can be difficult to locate, but farmers markets are becoming more common and you can even produce your own if you've got a green thumb.

WHAT ARE THE BENEFITS OF ORGANIC FOOD?

In a perfect world, we would all eat farm-to-table meals every day and eat all of our food from local, organic farmers. Nevertheless, who has the requisite resources to carry out such an undertaking?

If you want to reap the benefits of organic food, you don't have go "all in." In other cases, merely washing or peeling off the skin isn't enough to remove pesticide residues from food.

You can greatly limit your exposure to pesticides by opting for organic versus conventional for the following foods:

Produce such as celery, peaches, nectarines (imported), cucumbers, cherry tomatoes, and snap peas (imported), as well as potatoes, spicy peppers, and blueberries are all readily available in the United States and other countries across the globe.

The "Clean Fifteen" is a list of conventional foods that have the fewest pesticide residues and hence are less essential when deciding what to buy organic:

Cucumber, sweet corn (fresh or frozen), pineapple, pineapple chunks (frozen), onions, sweet pea pods (frozen), mangoes, papayas, kiwis, and sweet potatoes.

For this reason alone, switching to organic dairy is a good "investment," because the pesticides found in conventional animal feed end up in their milk. Pesticide residues can be found in conventional butter, whereas organic butter does not. 16

When it comes to eating meat, becoming organic is a smart option if you consume a lot of fatty foods.

HOW TO BUY ORGANIC FOOD FOR A CHEAP PRICE

When it comes to incorporating some organic foods into your diet, you're undoubtedly concerned about the cost, but that's understandable.

Even while organic goods are more expensive than their conventional equivalents, there are numerous ways to make the conversion more reasonable.

ENJOY YOUR FOOD WHEN IT'S IN SEASON

If you schedule your meals around what's in season, you won't be eating organic strawberries in the dead of winter, but you will save a lot of money on imported items.

SHOP BY THE POUND if possible.

Bulk sections in local organic co-ops and health food stores can save you a lot of money on staples like beans, grains, and spices, among other things.

If you buy in bulk during the season and can, dry, can, or freeze the food, you can save money by switching to organic co-ops and avoiding conventional store-bought items.

CHECK OUT RIPE FOODS FOR CHEAP OFFERS.

When it comes to food that is about to go bad, like spotted bananas, most health food stores provide an area just for those items.

It's a win-win situation because these meals are generally discounted and you may "cherry pick" the tastiest ones.

IF POSSIBLE, PURCHASE FROZEN

Research has shown that frozen foods are nutritionally similar to, and in some cases better than, fresh foods in terms of cost and convenience.

17

It's also helpful to remember this when stocking up on seasonal produce in large quantities. Blanch and freeze the remainder after you've used what you need!

Prepackaged foods should be avoided at all costs.

Remember that these organic "luxuries" come at a steep price, despite how easy and attractive the packaging may be.

You'll save money if you only buy whole foods that you have to cook and prepare yourself.

Whenever possible, select store brands.

Generic lines of organic food are available in many supermarkets and boutique stores, including organic fruit, pasta and grains, condiments, and more.

Generic items are far less expensive than their name-brand counterparts, but don't be fooled: they are held to the same farming and processing standards as the name brands.

THE FINAL ANALYSIS

There is no guarantee that eating organic will improve your health, but the advantages of eating organic foods are real and can be quite considerable in some situations.

Including organic foods in your diet may lessen your risk of disease and increase your lifespan, and that's well worth the additional cost!

There are no synthetic pesticides, genetically modified organisms (GMOs), petroleum- and sewage sludge-based fertilisers, or irradiation in organic crops.

It's important to note that organic cattle must be raised without the use of antibiotics, growth hormone or animal byproducts, and must have access to the outdoors as well as organic feed.

Organic food is better for you than regular food since it contains more nutrients.

Pesticides are less likely to be found in organic crops.

There are less antibiotic-resistant microorganisms in organic meats.

There are no growth hormones present in organic meats, which means they are safer for your health.

It's not necessary to go "all in" on organic if you don't want to. Pesticide residues are more concentrated in some foods than others (the "Dirty Dozen").

Since the pesticides in the grain that conventional cows eat end up in the milk, buying organic full-fat dairy is an excellent "investment."

Despite the fact that organic food is more expensive than conventional food, there are a number of ways to keep the cost down.

Chapter Five

HOW TO COOK

COOKING GREAT FOOD FOR THE MINIMALIST!

In a way, cooking is both a child's game and an adult's delight. Cooking is an act of love when it is done well. He is CRAIG CLAIBORNE

A common misconception about good cooking is that it takes a lot of skill and knowledge to pull it off.

Is there anything better than seeing a long line of rotisserie chickens waiting for hungry customers in a supermarket store? Roasting a chicken at home is a breeze, but did you know it's just as easy as sprinkling some spices on the bird and putting it in the oven?

Let's look at "ready-to-bake" foods like microwave dinners and the like. For the fifteen minutes it takes to prepare frozen pizza, you could have used that time to make a whole-food pie from scratch. The ingredients list demonstrates that they don't even qualify as food.

Real food and tasty food can be made easily, cheaply and quickly if you understand some fundamental cooking and food storage techniques.

Let's get started, shall we?

THE 12 MOST REPEATED MISTAKES IN THE KITCHEN

Most of us have no formal training in the art of cooking, and it's a real tragedy. We spend countless hours drilling arithmetic equations and sentence patterns, but we devote virtually no time to learning how to prepare nutritious meals for our families and our own bodies.

This means that many of us have succumbed to typical culinary blunders that make our meals more difficult to prepare and less pleasurable.

This is a list of the twelve most common blunders people make when writing.

TASTING AFTER YOU'VE FINISHED COOKING

Trying a new recipe and being let down by the taste is something we've all experienced at some point or another.

Keep in mind that since a recipe is based on the personal tastes of the author, the spice levels and flavours you like may differ from those listed. Culinary disasters can be avoided if you constantly taste your food while cooking.

Cooking, on the other hand, necessitates your constant attention in order to go from good to exceptional.

FAILING TO PREPARE IN ADVANCE

Those who are new to cooking tend to improvise while those who are more experienced prepare ahead to ensure that the dinner is as delightful as possible.

In this manner:

Get the motivation to eat healthfully.

Reminisce about the foods you ate as a child by reading food publications, browsing the internet, and looking at photos. Your thoughts will come to you easily. The more ideas you come up with, the better.

Draw up a menu

A simple menu of hot and cold dishes with a range of ingredients, flavours and textures may be drafted quickly..

Also, don't forget to keep things simple! The Tour de France is still a long way off for you.

Make a list of everything you need to buy and what you need to prepare.

Make a grocery list once you've settled on a menu and everything you'll need to buy is in place.

You'll need a list of what you're going to cook and when, starting with the dishes that take the longest to cook and ending with the ones that take the least (such as preparing a garnish).

It's also a good idea to "batching" your prep work, which means washing and peeling all of your vegetables at once.

When you should simmer, you're scalding.

Increasing the temperature of a dish to speed up the cooking process can result in a hazy, rough, or dry mess.

To achieve a simmer, set the stove to a temperature where a bubble breaks the surface every second or two.

You're putting yourself at risk if you go any further than that.

CONSIDERING THAT YOUR OVEN IS PERFECTLY WORKING

Most novice cooks aren't even aware that ovens might have uneven characteristics, such as hot or chilly regions.

To find yours, bake a single layer of bread on a cookie sheet for a few minutes at 350 degrees as part of the "bread test." Your oven's hot zones can be discovered by toasting the bread, allowing you to alter your baking methods in the future.

The bread in the back left corner of your oven may come out browner than the other pieces if you rotate your dishes while baking or place them in a more evenly heated region of the oven. Doing so will ensure that your food doesn't cook in hot regions.

Convection baking, on the other hand, uses hot air instead of heating components to cook the food. Faster cooking and even heating are two significant advantages of using a convection oven, as well as the elimination of cold patches.

When it comes to cooking meats, seafood, veggies, and other firm foods, convection baking is a great option.

ADDING FOOD TO A HOT PAN AFTER IT'S COOL.

A well-heated pan is essential when searing or sautéing because it prevents food from sticking and helps you get the desired crust or sear.

That "pssshhhhhhh" sound you're looking for is called "thermal shock," and it's what you want.

In order to test whether your pan is hot enough, dribble some water on it. It's not ready if there's no sizzle.

OVERFILLING YOUR PANEL WITH THINGS

Overcrowding your pan is the quickest way to lose the flavorful sizzle. Keep in mind that without searing, there will be no crust!

Make sure you cook your food in batches so that each piece gets the golden brown patina it deserves!

Improperly measuring ingredients

To be a competent cook, you don't need to measure to the microgram, but you do need to invest in suitable measuring cups and spoons for both dry and wet components.

Consider how you fill your utensils, as well. Using a 1-cup scoop to measure out sugar or flour will result in a lot more than the recipe calls for. As an alternative, use a knife to level the ingredient after it has been spooned into the cup.

TOO MUCH TURNING OF YOUR FOOD

It's a good time to be a lazy cook!

When cooking on the stove or grill, turning the meat too frequently can prevent it from developing a beautiful sear or breading coat. Instead, allow the meat to cook for the time specified in the recipe. It should only be turned once.

INABILITY TO READ THE TEMPERATURE OF MEAT

Using a meat thermometer is an essential tool for any novice chef.

Don't rely solely on appearances to determine the degree of completion. Cook your meat to a safe and acceptable temperature with the help of a digital thermometer.

Later in this chapter, we'll go through how to utilise a thermometer.

TOO MUCH SALT IN THE MARINADE OR BREADING

Pre-cooking seasoning is essential to guarantee that your meat gets the proper amount of salt.

While a high-sodium diet is common in the West, most individuals don't salt their food sufficiently to make it taste good (their sodium comes mainly from packaged foods).

Salt is a magical spice if you're looking for it. In the past, it was a highly prized and sought-after product. It's always a good idea to use a generous amount of salt when cooking.

Not Allowing Your Meat to Reach Room Temperature

If you cook a steak that's been sitting in the fridge for a while, the surface will be charred but the inside will be cold.

Before preparing your meats, leave them out on the counter for 15 to 30 minutes to get them up to room temperature. (Also, wipe the counter down completely before chopping vegetables on it.)

Components of poor quality are used.

High-quality beef can't be substituted for low-quality meat in the kitchen. When it comes to fresh vs. frozen and canned fruits and vegetables, this is the same. When compared to the previous, you may be amazed at how much better the latter tastes.

Always keep in mind that basic cooking methods combined with high-quality ingredients always outperform more complex methods and lower-quality ingredients.

The bottom line is that great food starts with wonderful ingredients, so invest as much money as you can afford in this area.

While the methods used to grow and harvest the food have a significant impact on the final product's quality, the way it is stored before cooking also has a significant impact.

Learn how to buy, store, and prepare a variety of animal proteins in the following paragraphs.

The basics of buying, storing, and preparing fish.

The health benefits of fish are well-known, but here's a short refresher.

In addition to being low in calories, high in protein, and rich in brain-boosting omega-3 fatty acids, fish is widely regarded as a "brain food" because of its high concentration of these vital fats.

More omega-3 fats in your diet can help keep your heart healthy.

One of the leading causes of death in the world is a heart attack, and omega-3 fatty acids have been shown to help prevent them.

1 When it comes to heart disease, those who consume one or more servings of fish each week are 15% less likely to develop the condition. 2

The cognitive deterioration of people who consume a lot of fish appears to be less rapid, according to research based on observation. A lower risk of type 1 diabetes in children, protection against vitamin D deficiency, and reduced risk of macular degeneration in women have all been associated to omega-3 consumption. 3

Because fish oil supplements have been demonstrated to boost muscle protein synthesis, reduce muscle soreness, and prevent weight gain, athletes should pay even more attention to fish.

4

To sum it up? Fish is a wonderful source of omega-3 fatty acids, and it's an easy method to get them.

FISH CAN BE PURCHASED SMARTLY.

Mercury content should be the first thing you look for when buying seafood.

Following these instructions from the Natural Resources Defense Council can help you reduce your intake of fish-based mercury.

5

You can eat these fish as often as you like because they have the lowest mercury content.

Anchovies, butterfish, caTFISH, crawfish, crawfish/crayfish, croaker (ATLANTIC), flounder, haddock (ATLANTIC), herring, Mackerel (N. ATLANTIC, CHUB), Mullet, PERCH (OCEAN), PLAICE, POLLOCK, SALMON (CANNED OR FRESH), SARDINE, SHAD (AMERICAN), SOLE (PACIFIC), TILAPIA, TROUT (FRESHWATER), WHITEFISH, and WHITING.

PER MONTH, PERSONS WITH MODERATE MERCURY CONTENT SHOULD EAT NO MORE THAN SIX SERVINGS OF THIS FISH.

CARP, CROAKER (WHITE PACIFIC), HALIBUT (ATLANTIC, PACIFIC), JACKSMELT (SILVERSIDE), LOBSTER, MONKFISH, SABLEFISH, SKATE, SNAPPER, TUNA (CANNED CHUNK LIGHT), TUNA (SKIPJACK), WEAKFISH (SEA TROUT)

THREE OR LESS SERVINGS PER MONTH WOULD BE A SAFE AMOUNT.

BOILER, GROUPER, MACKEREL (SPANISH, GULF), SEA BASS (CHILEAN), and TUNAFISH (YELLOWFIN)

It's best to avoid eating these fish at the same time because of their high mercury content.

TILEFISH, MARLIN, TUNA, ORANGE ROUGHY SHARK, TILEFISH, MARLIN (BIGEYE, AHI)

Aside from mercury content, you may notice claims like "wild caught" or "farm reared" fish when shopping for fish.

"Wild caught" may sound healthy, but the science is inconclusive.

Wild-caught and farm-raised fish have similar nutritional characteristics in terms of their nutrient content. Farm-raised trout, on the other hand, contain more vitamin A and selenium than wild-caught trout. However, the nutritional content of farmed and wild-caught rainbow trout is essentially comparable.

Farm-raised fish often have higher concentrations of the essential omega-3 fatty acids than wild-caught fish. For example, farmed Atlantic salmon has higher omega-3 fatty acids than wild Atlantic salmon.

Wild-caught vs. farm-raised fish is also less of a worry than many have made it out to be when it comes to pollutants.

Researchers in 2004 found ten times more possibly carcinogenic compounds in farmed fish than in their wild-caught counterparts in a study that caused quite a stir.

12 But despite the headlines, the level of contaminants in the water was still less than 2% of the amount considered harmful.

Further research has showed that farm-raised and wild-caught fish contain the same levels of pollutants.

13

The environmental impact of both farmed and wild-caught fish is hazy, as both involve unsustainable practises. The Monterey Bay Aquarium's Seafood Watch programme is an excellent resource for learning about the various threats facing different species of fish.

No matter what kind of fish you buy, whether wild-caught or farm-raised, remember these rules:

Purchase from a trusted source. Buying fish from a reputable local fish market rather than a big-box supermarket is more likely to yield a superior product.

Put fish through a sniffer test. The fragrance of fresh, unfrozen fish should be ocean or cucumber-like. Fish with an overpowering odour should be avoided.

You'll want to look for fish with supple skin. Try to poke a finger into the fish if you can. Fresh fish flesh will spring back to life. The fish is passed its peak if the indentation remains.

Observe the flesh for signs of moisture. The presence of a milky liquid on a fresh fish fillet indicates rot.

Examine the skin's texture. Scales should be shiny and smooth when buying skin-on fillets. There are several telltale signs of ageing, such as ruffled scales or a drab appearance.

As an alternative to buying fresh fish, you may be able to buy frozen fish, either locally or through an online supplier.

"Frozen-at-sea" (fas) labels are a good indicator. As soon as the fish is carried on board the ship, it is immediately flash-frozen, giving it a better flavour and quality than fish that has been treated longer.

Keep an eye out for freezer burns. The fish has lost moisture as a result of thawing and refreezing, as seen by white, dehydrated patches or visible ice crystals.

Moisture- and vapor-proof packaging should be sought out. Fish that have been packaged in this manner perform better than those that have been overwrapped.

FISH STORAGE IN THE RIGHT MANNER

Fresh fish should be cooked within 24 hours of purchase and any leftovers should be frozen. For up to two or three days, cooked fish can be kept in the refrigerator.

Store whole or filleted fish in packed ice to prevent moisture loss while it is being temporarily stored.

If the fat level is low, frozen fish can be stored for up to a year, depending on how long it has been frozen.

No longer than three months should fatty fish, such as mackerel and trout, be stored in the frozen state. Up to a year's worth of frozen lobster, shrimp, and scallops, as well as cod, flounder, and other lean fish, can be kept in the freezer.

Place frozen fish in the refrigerator and let it thaw for 18 to 24 hours per pound before cooking. Frozen fish can be thawed more quickly if necessary by running it under cold water.

FISH COOKING TECHNIQUES

With so many kinds of fish to choose from, even minimalist chefs have plenty of alternatives for preparing them to bring out the best in both their texture and flavour

For a wonderful meal, follow these simple tips:

Baking

Place the fish on a baking sheet that has been sprayed with cooking spray. For every inch of thickness, bake uncovered at 450° F for 10 minutes.

frying in a pan

Over medium to medium-high heat, warm a little amount of butter or oil. Seafood should be cooked for 4 to 5 minutes on each side.

Grilling

Place the oiled grill grate over the hot coals or gas flames, and close the cover. When using indirect heat, cook the seasoned fish for 15 minutes, or for 4 to 5 minutes on each side (per inch of thickness). Thicker pieces of fatty fish, or smaller fish that can be grilled in a basket, are preferred.

Poaching

Make sure the water or stock is just barely covering the seasoned fish in the pan. Cover and cook the fillets for 8 to 10 minutes at a low boil. Make a sauce using the leftover poaching liquid.

Microwaving

When in a hurry, a boneless fish fillet can be quickly and easily heated in the microwave. A microwave-safe dish with a thick section on one side is ideal for cooking fish. Portion out a tiny amount of liquid before adding the fish to the container. On high power, cook the meat for three minutes each pound, adding salt afterward.

If you don't have the time or willingness to prepare a whole recipe, you can make a tasty fish seasoning by combining the following components:

1 tablespoon of dried basil

1 tbsp. of dried rosemary crushed

Dry parsley: 1 tbsp

2 tbsp. of sea salt.

black pepper, ground, 2 tblsp

Dry oregano leaves (1 tsp)

Onion powder: 1 Tbsp

PURCHASE, STORAGE, AND COOKING SEASONED FISH

Aside from the B vitamins (such as B12), protein, iron, zinc, and other elements such as carnosine and creatine found in meat, a diet heavy in meat provides a number of other health benefits as well.

Though studies have shown processed meats might create health problems, this does not hold true for high-quality meat that you prepare yourself.

Here, you'll learn how to get the most out of your money using this part.

THE RIGHT WAY TO PURCHASE MEAT.

The most basic rule in meat shopping is: don't buy anything if it stinks.

In addition, it's easy to tell which meats are fresh and which aren't.

When it comes to red meat, the freshest pieces should be vivid red. The browning of red meat indicates that it has been exposed to the elements for a long period of time, and it should be avoided. Refrain from consuming vacuum-sealed meat that has developed air bubbles on the surface.

It is important to avoid odours and evident symptoms of ageing, like bruising or greenish spots, while purchasing fresh chicken. Additionally, it should have a smooth, non-slimy texture.

Local butcher shops, farmers markets, coops, and local farmers (who often offer "shares" of cows, pigs, and other animals) are the best places to buy "clean," chemical-free meat.

HOW TO STORE MEAT IN A SMARTER MANNER

Meat should be stored in accordance with these instructions from the USDA:

Raw poultry and ground beef should only be kept in the refrigerator for a maximum of one or two days at a temperature no higher than 40 degrees Fahrenheit. You can freeze the meat if you can't utilise it within this time frame.

Refrigerate raw beef, veal, lamb, and pork roasts, steaks, and chops for up to three to five days. Don't utilise what you can't freeze.

Meats and poultry should be stored in the refrigerator for no more than three to four days after they have been cooked.

If you plan on storing red meat or poultry in the freezer, you should do everything you can to keep the meat from being exposed to the elements.

If vacuum sealing is not an option, then place the meat in a zippered bag and cover it with aluminium foil before sealing it. In this manner, meat can be kept indefinitely.

Keep it in your fridge for 24 to 48 hours to thaw frozen red meat or poultry (longer if needed for larger cuts or roasts). Meat thawing on the counter can result in bacteria accumulating on the meat's exterior layers while the meat's interior remains frozen.

MEAT COOKING IN AN EFFICIENT MANNER

However, cooking times and temperatures must be adjusted for poultry and red meat in order to achieve the same results.

a red meat

Dry-heat cooking and wet-heat cooking are the two methods available for preparing red meat.

Grilling, broiling, sautéing, roasting, and stir-frying are all examples of dry-heat cooking.

Steaming, poaching, stewing, slow cooking, pot roasting, and braising are examples of wet-heat cooking procedures.

Steaks, which are naturally tender, should be cooked using dry heat methods and shorter cooking periods as a general rule.

It takes longer, slower cooking times with moist heat methods to melt the collagen and elastin in roasts, which have a higher concentration of these connective tissues than steaks.

Poultry

Depending on the cut of poultry, any or all of these methods can be used to prepare it.

Whole chickens, on the other hand, are a more economical alternative to buying individual chicken breasts, though the larger size necessitates more time spent in the kitchen during preparation.

In contrast, thin chicken breast fillets must be closely maintained to avoid drying out.

Meat Thermometer Reminders

When we talked about the necessity of using a good meat thermometer earlier in this chapter, did you recall?

And this tip deserves its own section.

Your meat thermometer should be placed in the following spot:

It's as though you've got a steak with two different thicknesses. It's likely that the thin end of the steak will cook faster than the thick end if you grill it for 20 minutes and then insert a meat thermometer.

Getting the positioning of your meat thermometer just right is as vital as the temperature to which you prepare your food.

Poultry

For a full chicken or turkey, the inner thigh near the breast but not touching the bone is where you should take a reading. If your bird is stuffed, take a thermometer to the stuffing and make sure it's a temperature of 165 degrees or higher. Individual chicken breasts should be measured at their thickest point.

meats such as lamb, veal, and mutton

Keep the thermometer away from bone, fat, and gristle by inserting it into the thickest section of the meat.

Meat minced

The thickest section of the dish shouldn't touch the serving dish when using ground beef or poultry in a dish like meatloaf or casserole. If you're working with ground beef patties, try inserting the meat thermometer from the side.

You're seeking for what kind of temperature.

At this point, your meat thermometer should read between 140 and 160 degrees Fahrenheit, depending on the type of thermometer you're using.

Rest Your Strength.

You'll sacrifice some of the juicy, soft flavour of your meat if you consume it right away after it comes out of the stove, oven, or grill.

It's because the cooking process concentrates the meat's juices in the centre of the animal, making the rest tough and dry. After a few minutes of rest, the juices that have been trapped inside of the cut will seep out and "rehydrate" it.

This is a guide on seasoning food for the minimalist.

Unseasoned chicken breast isn't anything to write home about, as anyone who's ever eaten it can attest.

Even a pinch of salt and a grind of black pepper can transform a nice piece of red meat into something extraordinary.

A lot more may be done to make beef truly exceptional.

SALT

As long as anyone can remember, we've been told that we need to cut back on our salt intake.

In the early 1900s, French doctors claimed that six of their patients with high blood pressure also ate a high-salt diet.

Concerns about high blood pressure were heightened in the 1970s when Lewis Dahl of the Brookhaven National Laboratory fed rats a diet containing 500 grammes of sodium daily, inducing hypertension in the rodents (for comparison, the average U.S. adult consumes 3.4 grammes of sodium daily).

Dahl further stated that countries like Japan, which consume a lot of sodium in their food, have greater rates of hypertension and stroke.

As a result of his findings, as well as his foundation for fearing sodium, has began to disintegrate This elemental chemical may not be as toxic as originally thought, according to recent study.

"There is no evidence for long-term benefit from limiting salt intake" was the conclusion of an exhaustive assessment of the sodium literature published in 2003.

14

More than 6,250 people from seven studies were included in a meta-analysis eight years later, which confirmed the findings of the original study and concluded that lowering salt is not an effective way to lower the risk of heart attack, stroke, or death in those with normal or high blood pressure.

15

Another study from 2015 found a link between a lower sodium intake and an increased risk of death from heart disease.

16

Would it be prudent to limit your salt intake? When it comes to lowering blood pressure, preventing strokes and heart disease, is it really vital to limit your intake of sodium?

We do know that sodium is required for our bodies to operate, even if the science behind it isn't quite obvious. In order to maintain the proper balance of intracellular and extracellular fluids, sodium binds and transports water throughout the body.

In addition, we know that genetics and culture play a role. Some people are more sensitive than others to salt.

In the end, this is what matters:

Salt-related issues are rare as long as you're not consuming a lot of pre-packaged or highly processed meals or if you have a bizarre obsession with over-salting every meal you eat.

That being said, let's move on to salt and cooking.

When it comes to flavouring your food, salt is the most vital. The flavour of meat and fish can be enhanced by a pinch of salt. Is also a great complement to many other kinds of herbs and spices.

You should try a variety of salts to see what works best for you.

While all three types of salt have distinct flavours, they may all be used in a variety of ways, from brining to rubbing to seasoning.

When it comes to adding salt, be slow and steady. Season in little amounts throughout the cooking process, using a bowl of salt on the counter as a reminder.

Unless you're adding salty items like bacon or capers, you should always add salt to a pot of simmering soup.

If you overdo it, what will happen?

It's no problem at all. There are several ways to soften the flavours, such as adding a little milk or unsalted butter. Grated raw potatoes, cooked in a salty broth for seven to eight minutes before being strained, is a Julia Child technique that some cooks swear by.

Temperature and time will also affect the saltiness of your cuisine. Let's say you're in the mood for ham. Because it's cold, ham tastes saltier than when it's heated, where its flavour becomes more savoury, it's best served cold. The method of salting a ham dish varies depending on the recipe and how it will be served.

A day or two after cooking, you might notice that leftovers have a different flavour character when you take them out of the fridge. The saltiness of a dish that was previously overpowering may have subsided, while other flavour combinations may have the opposite effect. A smart suggestion is to taste and adjust the amount of salt before serving your leftovers.

In fact, it's a terrific method to see how much salt you're adding and distribute it more evenly across the dish by tossing the salt from a height of 10 to 12 inches.

ACIDS

Acids and bases are on opposite sides of the pH scale, as you may recall from high school chemistry. Chemically speaking, acids are simply molecules that are capable of losing their hydrogen ion, and this is what gives them their characteristic flavour characteristics such as tartness and acidity.

Acids like vinegar, lemon juice, and lime juice are used by professional chefs to enhance savoury or sweet dishes.

Some red wine vinegar, for example, can enhance the flavour of your beef stew, while lemon juice can brighten up your fruit salad.

Using acids to modify the structure of proteins can be used to cook food in some cases. Even though no heat has been applied, pickled eggs can be regarded "cooked" because of the vinegar's acidity, despite not having been heated.

Acids can be used in a variety of ways, but their most common use is in the presentation of food. Pour a bit of lemon or lime juice over your dish when you're done cooking and it will bring out the best in your food!

Acids are essential to marinades, as well.

You won't be able to get much flavour out of a tough cut of meat if you merely slap on your seasonings. If you add an acid like vinegar, tomato juice, or citrus juice to your spices, they'll be more effective in penetrating the meat's outermost layers because of the protein-altering actions.

Vinaigrette dressings can also benefit from the addition of acids. For salad dressing, mix one part acid with three parts oil and add spices or seasonings as desired. The possibilities are truly unlimited if you tweak the ratio and mix up your additions.

However, don't worry about adding acids to your recipes; they're easy to incorporate. If you overdo it, you can rebalance the meal by adding sugar or oil, depending on the recipe you're using.

SEASONINGS AND INGREDIENTS

The variety of spices and seasonings accessible to you is only surpassed by the diversity of cuisines. It is possible to take the same ingredients in an entirely different direction with each spice combination.

Cooking a chicken breast with bell peppers in a wok is a good example. Asian, jerk, or even Italian flavours can be included into the dish using various spice and ingredient combinations.

Incorporate fresh, ground, and whole spices into your dishes as you go through the process of experimenting with different flavours.

All spices that are "warm": cardamom, nutmeg, cinnamon, curry, turmeric

Flavors deemed "hot" include cayenne pepper, red pepper flakes, Sriracha, and Tabasco sauce.

Basil, parsley, sage, rosemary, tarragon, mint, and thyme are all examples of "green" flavours.

Garlic, garlic powder, onion powder, scallion, mustard, and horseradish are all "pungent" flavours.

'Zesty' flavours include ginger, orange and lemon zest.

Diced bacon and smoked salt are also included in the "smoky" flavour profile.

Walnuts, sesame, soy, pecans, and pistachios are all "nutty" flavours.

Sugar, molasses, maple syrup, honey, and other "sweet" flavours

Avoid "dead" herbs and spices, as well. Check the "use by" dates on your products on a regular basis and replace any that have passed their expiration date. Spices and herbs can also be checked for freshness by smelling them. There is no flavour in your food if you don't have any fragrance. When in doubt, it's best to toss them.

Grow your own spices and herbs if you want the best quality.

Many culinary herbs can be easily cultivated in pots in kitchen windowsills. Once they are harvested, simply trim the stems and store them upright, covered with a plastic bag, in the refrigerator, just like fresh flowers.

The timing of when you add your herbs and spices to the dish is important, too.

It is best to add delicate and subtle fresh herbs like oregano, basil, and tarragon right before serving, after the food has finished cooking. Dry herbs on the other hand, on the other hand, have a powerful flavour and can be easily dispersed during cooking. Incorporate them at the start.

CPSIA information can be obtained
at www.ICGtesting.com
Printed in the USA
LVHW061208190722
723853LV00014B/556

9 781804 768884